The Human Body Handbook

A Simple Yet Powerful Guide to Maximizing Your
Health and Function So You Can Avoid Drugs and
Surgery, and Live a Longer, Healthier, More Active Life

Alex Wiant DC

To the humans of planet Earth, so you may live longer, healthier and higher quality lives.

The Great American Health Tragedy

The state of health in the US is at an all time low. We spend over $9,000 per person per year on health care, and have virtually the same life expectancy as someone in Cuba (79.8 years vs 79.4 years), who spends only $300 per year on health care.

We are over doctored, over medicated, and all this spending isn't making us healthier. In fact, the reliance on modern medicine is not only making us sicker, it is killing us.

In our insurance driven model of health care, people don't get concerned about their health until they start feeling bad or looking bad - showing signs or symptoms of disease. Only then do you go to the doctor to get medicine or surgery, which doesn't address the cause of your disease, it only covers it up or cuts it out to give you the illusion of health.

Even if you go for a once a year physical exam, the screening procedures you might go through only catch diseases when they have already progressed to the point you have serious detectable disease.

This is not the way to good health.

If you don't get concerned about your health until you start looking bad or feeling bad, you are susceptible to the top three killers in the US: **Heart disease, cancer, and medical errors.**

Can you feel fine and have a fatal heart attack? Sure. Can you have stage four cancer and not know it? Of course. Can you go to the hospital and die from a medical mistake? Yeah. <u>More than 400,000 per year die from preventable harm to patients.</u>[1]

Having health insurance is great, but it doesn't mean you are healthy.

Health insurance is just like any other insurance: protection against a catastrophic event. You have fire insurance to protect against fire, flood insurance to protect against flood. If you live in a flood plain, your flood insurance is going to be higher than someone who lives on a mountain, because you have a higher chance of flood.

If you contract a disease, are in a car accident, or sever a leg, insurance will be there to bail you out. Insurance does not exist to keep you healthy. Insurance doesn't pay for your regular gym membership, it doesn't pay for you to eat healthy food, and it doesn't pay for you to manage a healthy lifestyle.

Health insurance *insures* your health. It doesn't **ensure** it.

Ensuring your health involves taking care of your body on a regular basis and not basing your health on an absence of symptoms or how you look or how you feel.

Ensuring your health involves maximizing the <u>function</u> of your body, which is exactly what this book is about.

This book reveals exactly how to:

• Naturally boost your healing ability by reducing and eliminating stress

• Avoid joint pain and replacement surgeries by minimizing joint wear and tear

[1] James, John T. 2013. "A New, Evidence-Based Estimate of Patient Harms Associated with Hospital Care:" *Journal of Patient Safety* 9 (3): 122–28. doi:10.1097/PTS.0b013e3182948a69.

• Maintain your youth and vitality by keeping your muscles supple and youthful

• Reduce heart disease by maximizing heart and lung function

• Prevent diabetes and clogged arteries by eating the right kind of foods

• Live a longer, healthier, higher quality life by significantly lower your risk factors

This book explains how physical, chemical and emotional stress impacts our bodies and outlines steps we can take to reduce these effects, simply and easily.

Your body is a complex biological machine, and like any high performance precision instrument, it needs regular care and attention to function properly.

Everyone should have good health. Virtually everyone can.

See you inside.

Chapter 1: The Nervous System, Your Body's Electrical System

Your nervous system is the single most important system in the body. This communication superhighway begins with your body's central organizing authority, the central nervous system (CNS), which includes the brain and spinal cord. The central nervous system interacts with the body through the peripheral nervous system (PNS).

Your brain is made up of over 400 billion cells, a quarter of which, over 100 billion, are actual nerve cells called neurons. Each neuron is in contact with, or synapses with thousands of other neurons, creating a communication network whose total connections reaches into the trillions, and whose total operational capacity can be quadrillions of operations per second.

All your senses, smell, taste, hearing, vision, and touch; all your conscious thought processes; all your body functions like breathing and heart beat; immune function like cell and tissue repair and regeneration; and all of your movement, balance and coordination are organized by this three pound central processing unit.

The CNS talks to our body through our peripheral nervous system. We interface with our muscles through our somatic nervous system, and our bodily functions are controlled by the autonomic nervous system.

The autonomic nervous system is broken into two parts, sympathetic and parasympathetic. These systems keep each other in balance. Generally, the way these systems work is when one is stimulated, the other is inhibited.

The sympathetic nervous system is responsible for handling emergencies and tasks that require immediate response. You may have heard of the fight or flight response. This is your sympathetic nervous system's job. It mobilizes parts of your body that help you through crisis situations. It controls the release of adrenaline and other substances which speed up your heart, open the airways into your lungs, shunt blood to your muscles from your skin and gut, initiate the production of blood sugar from your storage reserves for quick energy, and stop unnecessary bodily activities like digestion mediated by the parasympathetic nervous system.

The parasympathetic nervous system is responsible for rest and relaxation. It mediates digestion, controls head and face function like saliva and tear production, and controls urination and defecation.

Stress is a Killer

The sympathetic nervous system acts up in the presence of environmental stressors. Back in the day, it would be a flash of an orange tiger, seeing a child in danger, or zeroing in on prey. Today it is emotional stress from your mortgage or debt, or from traffic in the morning, chemical stress from environmental toxins, drugs or an unhealthy diet, or physical stress like gravitational pull, trauma, pain, and repetitive stress injuries.

All these physical, chemical and emotional stressors in our environment affect our nervous system. These stressors change the way our nervous system is able to adapt and respond to our internal and external environment.

A pioneer in stress research, Dr. Hans Sellye MD, came up with a term to define the physiological responses to stress, the General Adaptation Syndrome, or GAS. The GAS describes three stages of stress response: alarm, resistance, and recovery / exhaustion.

The problem is that most of us are under a constant barrage of stressors, don't have adequate time to recover, and are chronically in the exhausted state.

Internally, having a high level of constant stress and constant sympathetic activity lowers your immune function. Studies have shown that wounds take longer to heal and normal immune function against infections disease is suppressed when under stress.[2,3] This would be a reasonable response if you were truly in danger, as survival would be a priority.

However, in our stressed out world, this is a recipe for disease and dysfunction. Stress accelerates aging at the molecular level,[4] and according to various online health authorities including the CDC and WebMD, up to 95% of doctor visits are due to stress-related illnesses and diseases.

Conditions like anxiety, chronic fatigue, depression, mental disorders like bipolar disorder, Alzheimer's and Parkinson's, and other illnesses can be worsened by stress induced immune decline.

---

[2] Segerstrom, Suzanne C. and Miller, Gregory E.: Psychological Stress and the Human Immune System: A Meta-Analytic Study of 30 Years of Inquiry. Psychological Bulletin, Vol 130(4), Jul 2004, 601-630.

[3] Gouin JP. and Kiecolt-Glaser JK.: The impact of psychological stress on wound healing: methods and mechanisms. Immunol Allergy Clin North Am 2011; 31:81

[4] Epel, Elissa S., Elizabeth H. Blackburn, Jue Lin, Firdaus S. Dhabhar, Nancy E. Adler, Jason D. Morrow, and Richard M. Cawthon. 2004. "Accelerated Telomere Shortening in Response to Life Stress." *Proceedings of the National Academy of Sciences of the United States of America* 101 (49): 17312–15. doi:10.1073/pnas.0407162101.

Many of these patterns, especially when considering mental health, become self-perpetuating and worsen over time. These patterns become grooves, reinforced neural circuits, just like a well-rehearsed golf swing or baseball pitch.

A very simplified example of this might be someone who is depressed and avoids social interaction, but whose isolation will cause them to become more depressed and further avoid social contact.

Combating Stress

The following are easy and effective ways to combat stress:

Exercise

The three exercises everyone should be doing are resistance training, cardiovascular exercise (more on that later), and some form of enjoyable physical fun - something you can look forward to like golf, dancing, softball, any kind of physical activities you like. It is crucial to incorporate all three. Resistance training through your full range of motion to keep your muscles and joints healthy, cardiovascular exercise to ensure a strong heart and lungs, and physical fun, since for many people resistance training and doing cardio is a chore, it's important to have something fun to look forward to!

Prayer or meditation / Focused relaxation

Having the ability to clear your mind of racing thoughts is an important but difficult skill to develop. Meditation has been shown to reduce beta brainwaves - synonymous with active, anxious and conscious thinking, and increase alpha brainwaves - waves consistent with a state of relaxation. If you practice it you will enjoy less anxiety, less stress, fewer racing thoughts, a higher sense of wellbeing, and a host of other benefits.

There are many different ways to meditate, however the most simple way to start is by finding a comfortable place to sit or lay down, and for two to five minutes put all your attention on your breath. Breathe in through your nose for four seconds, then out for four seconds. If you notice your mind starting to wander, put it back on your breath. With time you will get better and be able to clear your head quickly and for longer periods of time. I like to do this before bed. It makes falling asleep much easier.

Having time dedicated to an activity that demands significant focus and concentration can also help reduce stress and force you to still a racing mind. Shooting guns and playing golf forces me to concentrate and free my mind of worries and anxieties. I know many people enjoy practicing yoga for the same benefits.

Proper rest

Getting adequate sleep is incredibly important to combat stress. This is the most obvious way to ensure an adequate recovery phase and prevent exhaustion. Incorporating exercise and prayer or meditation into your day will prime you for better sleep, as will the following guidelines:

To get the best sleep, you should avoid watching television for a few hours before bed. Ideally you shouldn't even have a television in the bedroom. The quickly moving pictures on TV and in movies attract your attention and actually prevent you from relaxing. Further, keep your bedroom free of clutter, electronics, exercise equipment, and definitely do not bring any work materials into the bedroom. Having them around will just remind you of work and change your frame of mind. Also, don't eat within three to four hours of sleep.

Most importantly, invest in a good mattress. A good mattress is the most important piece of furniture you can buy, and is worth spending some decent money on.

There is no other purchase you can make that will improve your quality of life and cost less to use than a mattress. If you wake up sore or uncomfortable or toss and turn at night, you owe it to yourself to invest in a new mattress. Don't be afraid to spend a few thousand dollars. Like I mentioned there is nothing you could buy that will cost less to use than a mattress. If you spend $5,000 on a mattress, keep it for 20 years and sleep eight hours a night, it will cost you 8.5 cents an hour to use. I don't think there is anything you can buy that gives you a better bang per buck than a great mattress.

I have an Intellibed. Intellibed relieves more pressure than any other mattress on the market, while providing excellent support. Intellibeds do not expel toxic gasses like many other mattresses, and are guaranteed for 30 years. They sell for a very fair price as well. It is by far the best bed I have slept in, and the best purchase I have ever made.

Visiting a chiropractor

Physically, high levels of stress cause muscle tightness, which then prevents proper joint function. Spasmed muscles and stuck joints can cause pain and further increase stress, causing more muscle tightness and more joint dysfunction. These situations compound by feeding the brain incorrect position information, creating error prone, self-perpetuating feedback loops.

Down the line, these dysfunctional joints can experience increased wear and tear, become arthritic and degenerative, cause more pain that increases your stress, and significantly reduce your quality of life.

A chiropractor's sole and unique objective is to detect and correct these poorly functioning joints. In chiropractic lingo, these dysfunctional joints are known as "subluxations."

When a chiropractor finds a subluxation, the chiropractor will put a quick force into the joint, known as a chiropractic adjustment, which frees the joint and allows for proper function. Resetting the joint forces the muscles around the joint to relax.

After getting adjusted, people often report a reduction in stress. This is proven, measurable, and occurs on many levels. The decrease in stress leaves them feeling relaxed and patients typically sleep much more soundly after getting adjusted.

Further, getting adjusted bombards the brain with new information. When joints move, nerve cells in the joint called mechanoreceptors send new movement and position information to the brain. This huge bombardment of information, plus considering that every brain cell synapses with 1000 or more other neurons, creates the equivalent of fireworks in the brain.

This effect functions as a pattern interrupt, breaking the current neurological brain pattern, and forcing the CNS into a parasympathetic state, as evidenced by research on how chiropractic adjustments affect brainwaves. Chiropractic puts patients into a predominantly alpha brainwave pattern, which is associated with relaxation and healing. The chiropractic adjustment also increases the general level of brainwave activity.[5]

Mental Health and Well Being

Dementia is a large topic of interest these days with the aging baby boomer population. One good rule of thumb to follow to keep a sharp mind is: use it or lose it! As people age typically they exercise less and receive less mental stimulation. Both exercise and mental stimulation are critical for brain fitness.

As we mentioned earlier, each neuron synapses with thousands if not tens of thousands of other neurons. Exercise stimulates sensory and motor areas of your brain, and has even been shown to increase nerve growth factor.[6]

Practicing movements with both sides of your body, like throwing, kicking, even brushing our teeth and combing our hair can create new motor patterns and new neural pathways in the brain.

You are never too old to explore new activities. Shooting baskets, playing golf, ballroom dancing and new forms of movement in general can keep your brain stimulated and reduce the possibility of dementia.

Varying mental stimulation is also a great way to stay sharp. Learning a second language has shown to delay dementia

[5] Barwell, R., Long, A., Byers, A., Schisler, C.: The effect of the Chiropractic adjustment on the brain wave pattern as measured by QEEG. Summarizing an additional 100 (approximately) cases over a three year period. The Chiropractic Journal, Jun 2008

[6] Russo-Neustadt, A. A., R. C. Beard, Y. M. Huang, and C. W. Cotman. 2000. "Physical Activity and Antidepressant Treatment Potentiate the Expression of

and recent studies have found that maintaining an active social life can cut cognitive decline by 70%.[7]

Using all your senses, listening to music, visiting new places and creating new experiences can stimulate the production of nerve growth factor. Doing puzzles like Sudoku, playing games that involve planning ahead and strategy like chess, and even simple childhood games like Memory all stimulate the brain, as does reading and writing.

The amazing communication system is so important that nature created a protective armor around it, the skull and spine. While the tissues outside our central nervous system can readily regenerate and repair, the only cells in your body that can't regenerate, are the ones in our brain and spinal cord, which is why they are so protected.

As you age, failing aspects of your spine can negatively affect this communication network and cause disease and dysfunction, making the health and function of your spine and skeleton, and the function of the nervous system and thereby the entire body INEXTRICABLY linked.

[7]James, Bryan D., Robert S. Wilson, Lisa L. Barnes, and David A. Bennett. 2011. "Late-Life Social Activity and Cognitive Decline in Old Age." Journal of the International Neuropsychological Society 17 (06): 998–1005. doi:10.1017/S1355617711000531.

Chapter 2: The Skeletal System

The skeleton is made of 206 bones and floats in a network of muscle and connective tissue known as fascia. Bones connect to other bones with ligaments and cartilage, and muscles connect to bone with tendons.

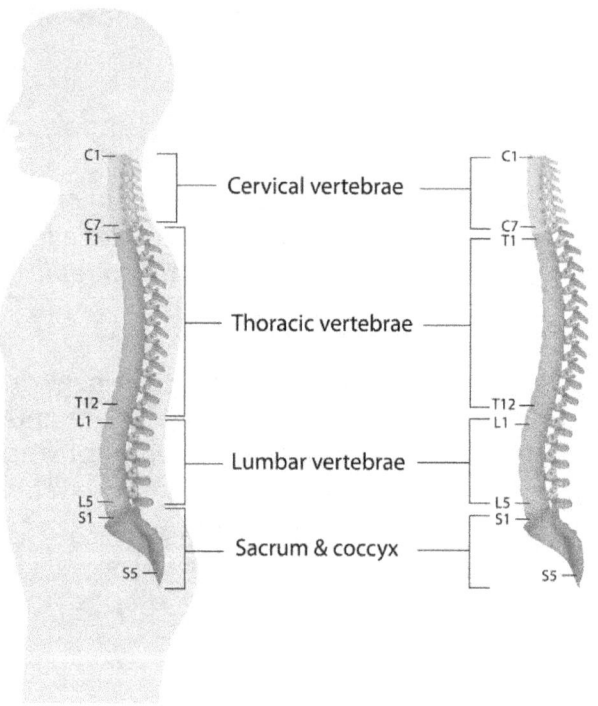

The spine is made up of 24 bones called vertebrae, and is broken into three sections, our cervical spine (neck), thoracic spine (mid and upper back) and lumbar spine (lower back). Each section has a corresponding curve. Each bone is separated by a shock absorbing cartilaginous disc, and is connected to its neighboring vertebrae with muscles and ligaments. Our spinal cord travels through all these bones, and at every joint, nerves exit to supply part of our body with the brain-body connection we need to function properly.

The joints that connect our vertebrae allow us to be flexible, but this flexibility can cause instability, and as we mentioned earlier, physical, chemical and emotional stressors in our environment can cause our muscles to tighten. These tight muscles prevent proper joint movement, which affects nerve function and communication, and can lead to significant dysfunction down the line.

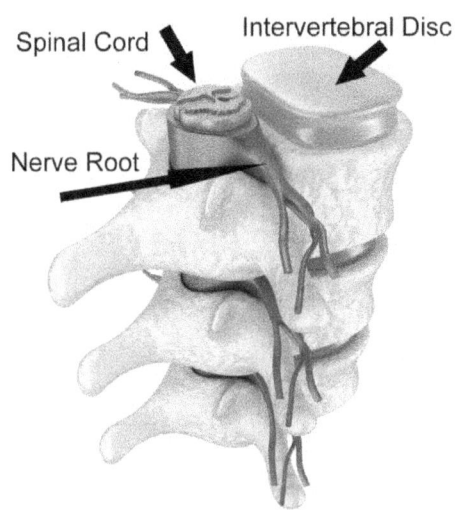

Spinal Cord

Intervertebral Disc

Nerve Root

Your Suspension System

You have 26 bones in your feet. It's imperative you support your feet with good shoes in order to keep all your other joints healthy. People with lower arches or flat feet really need to take extra care to wear supportive shoes. When your arches aren't supported and collapse, your tibia and femur (leg bones) will rotate, affect the alignment of your pelvis and create compensation in your entire spine. When your spine is not properly supported or aligned, the muscles that surround the spine can't function with even resting muscle tension and you will begin to develop muscle imbalances which ultimately lead to joint dysfunction and increased rates of degeneration.

Much to the chagrin of my clients usually the best shoes aren't that fashionable, although there are some exceptions, and high heels definitely aren't great for your feet or body. Flats are becoming increasingly popular these days however for many people they are completely inappropriate, because they don't provide any arch support. Further womens' flats squish the toes together and prevent the toes from splaying out like they should.

When you wear shoe with heels, even slight heels like virtually all running shoes and dress shoes, you are forced to compensate for the heel lift by maintaining tension in your calves and quads, otherwise you will fall forward. These changes in muscle tension encourage poor posture and contribute to the common muscle imbalances I go into a little later. Heels also cause bunions.

Four Critical Things to Look for in a Shoe

• Zero heel toe drop. The heel and toe should be on the same plane, essentially a "flat" shoe, except with arch support.

• Arch support. Some is better than none. If you have really flat feet, some custom insoles would likely benefit you.

• Wide toe box. This is crucial. You want your toes to be able to spread out when you walk, not be scrunched together.

• Cushioning. Your feet need some cushioning. If you walk all the time or run in shoes with no cushion, you will have a higher likelihood of causing stress fractures, which wearers of the Five Finger Toe Shoes quickly discovered.

The shoes I like best and wear the most are Merrell barefoot style shoes. I have gone through many pairs of Merrell Barefoot style shoes, and everyone who's bought a pair off my recommendation loves them. I urge you to buy a pair and wear them when you can.

I understand footwear is important as a fashion statement, and you may need to wear certain shoes for certain events, however when possible wear shoes that adhere to the four elements above. Foot health is critical to your skeletal and joint health, and further, a lot of our balance and coordination is managed by position data sent from our feet.

The 26 bones in our feet are all connected with joints and continuously send information to the brain about foot position. Scrunching the toes up and wearing high heels puts you in a position where your brain is not getting the adequate information it needs to properly coordinate your balance, not only from your feet, but by the rest of your joints above your feet which now have altered mechanics. Over time as permanent changes and adaptations occur in your feet and body, you are really going to handicap your ability to function.

If you fancy yourself an athlete or desire to function at your peak of balance and stability, you need to take care of your feet, and the easiest way to do that is by getting some barefoot style shoes with arch support, good cushioning and a wide toe box.

How Our Body Controls Balance, Posture and Coordination

Your body is constantly sending position information to the cerebellum, the portion of the brain responsible for motor control. This information allows us to maintain our balance and coordination, negotiate varying terrain in our environment, and stay upright on your two feet. It does this through proprioception.

Proprioception is a Latin word for "individual" or "one's own" perception, meaning perception of one's self or sense of ourselves. Your brain interprets your position through nerves in your joints and muscles.

In your joints these nerve cells are called mechanoreceptors and constantly transmit information regarding joint location and joint position. In your muscles, these cells are called muscle spindles and are constantly communicating your muscle length and muscle stretch.

Your brain processes this information from your joints and muscles to keep you balanced. When you are standing, for example, when you sway or shift your weight around, the brain detects this sway and shift through joint movement and subsequent change in muscle length. Your brain will respond by slightly tightening the stretching muscles to keep your body balanced and upright.

This ability of your brain to integrate our environment with our motor response is called "sensori-motor integration," and is considerably increased when all the joints in your spine and body are functioning properly.

Errors in the Computer

Now, past traumas like car accidents and falls can misalign your spine and damage support tissues like muscles, tendons and ligaments, compromising the body's sensori-motor integration.

Even muscle spasms from sudden or rapid change in position or chronically bad posture can cause joints to become stuck and send incorrect information to the brain, compromising the brain's ability to respond accurately to your surroundings.

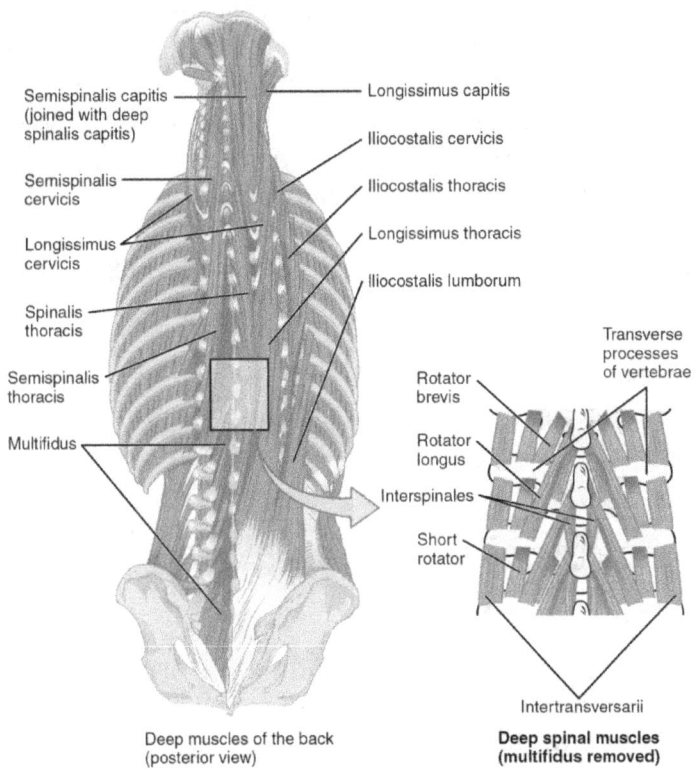

The small, delicate muscles of the spine along with the joints themselves send position information to the brain.

When your central nervous system isn't getting all the information it needs to make split second balance and coordination decisions, your ability to stay balanced and upright is compromised.

Additionally, movements requiring precision like a golf swing or tennis serve, or dribbling a ball down the field won't be as accurate without this information.

This is one of the reasons many athletes choose to be checked and adjusted on a regular basis. They know their brain needs all the information it can get about body position to increase body awareness and coordination, and decrease the possibility for rolling an ankle on the football field or losing their balance on a balance beam.

Non-athletes can significantly benefit from increased body awareness as well.

If you were clumsy in the past, or have a clumsy child, it's probable that errors in joint position sense contribute to the clumsiness.

In the elderly, stuck joints and poor body awareness can lead to increased falls, which in advanced age can be truly catastrophic.

In fact, there have been many studies performed that show how increasing joint position sense in the elderly with chiropractic care increases their stepping speed, reaction time, and can help prevent falls and lost balance.

Not only can stuck joints create errors in joint position sense and body response, they also cause pain.

When joints stop moving properly and cease sending position information, they allow nociceptors (pain nerves) to become activated which fire off pain signals. The associated spasmed muscles also send pain signals to the brain. Pain is like the check engine light coming on in our car. It says "Hey! Something's wrong!"

For optimal function, these joints need to be moving properly all the time. The only way to ensure all these joints are functioning properly is with chiropractic.

When stuck and not moving in the correct range of motion, or when the discs that separate our vertebrae become dry and begin to degenerate, increased stress on our vertebrae will cause disc bulges and bone spurs which can pinch nerves exiting the spine and even the spinal cord itself.

Disc Bulges

The discs between our vertebrae have a soft center that does the actual cushioning. This soft center is called the nucleus pulposus, and is like the jelly in a jelly donut. When the joint is stuck out of alignment, instead of having the weight distributed evenly over the disc, pressure will be concentrated in one area. If you imagine stepping on a jelly donut, this extra pressure will squeeze the soft center to one side. If there is enough pressure, the jelly will squeeze out and cause a herniated disc, which typically means it is surgery time.

If you keep the discs healthy through chiropractic adjustments, movement and exercise, you can significantly reduce the possibility of disc injury.

Disc Degeneration

Over 60% of people over 40 years of age have degenerating discs. When we are young and growing, we have a blood supply to our discs that provides nutrients and keeps them hydrated and healthy. By the time we reach maturity, the blood supply to our discs deteriorates, and at this point the only way to keep the discs hydrated is through motion.

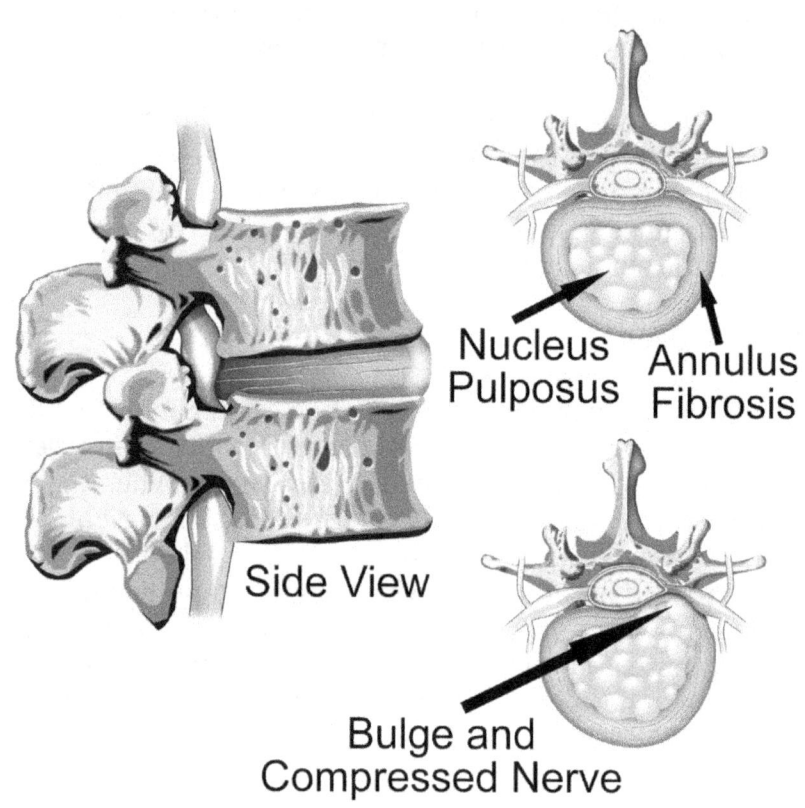

Nucleus Pulposus   Annulus Fibrosis

Side View

Bulge and Compressed Nerve

When the spine is moving properly, there is a pumping action in our joints and discs that keeps them hydrated by imbibing or absorbing moisture from surrounding tissues. This is the same action that causes a dry sponge to rehydrate, and a raisin to swell when dropped in water.

Over time, when the spine is not functioning or moving properly, these discs dry out and lose their shock absorbing properties. They become hard and increase the stress and pressure on our vertebrae. You have probably heard how a broken bone will heal to be stronger than it was before. It's true. A bone responds to stress by reinforcing itself and forming a callous. On our skin a callous is formed with thicker and harder skin. On a bone, a callous is formed with calcium deposits. This bony growth is known as a bone spur.

When disc degeneration occurs, growing bone spurs will physically pinch nerves by growing into the areas where nerves exit our spine. Bone spurs will even grow enough to fuse the spine together, essentially forming one bone, significantly reducing motion, function and health.

When you get to this level of degeneration it is game over.

Your body will not be able to manage your balance and coordination well, and communication between your brain and body will be significantly reduced, due to the degenerating spine putting permanent pressure on your nerves and spinal cord.

Not only will the nerves to our muscles be affected, but virtually all nerves will have reduced function from spinal degeneration. This reduction in nerve communication will compromise the ability of cells and tissues to adequately repair and regenerate leading to organ dysfunction, disease, and incontinence. One preventable cause of incontinence is stenosis, which is the narrowing of the spinal canal, and directly related to spine dysfunction and degeneration. The good news is there are ways to keep your spine healthy.

The best way to keep your spine healthy is by visiting a chiropractor.

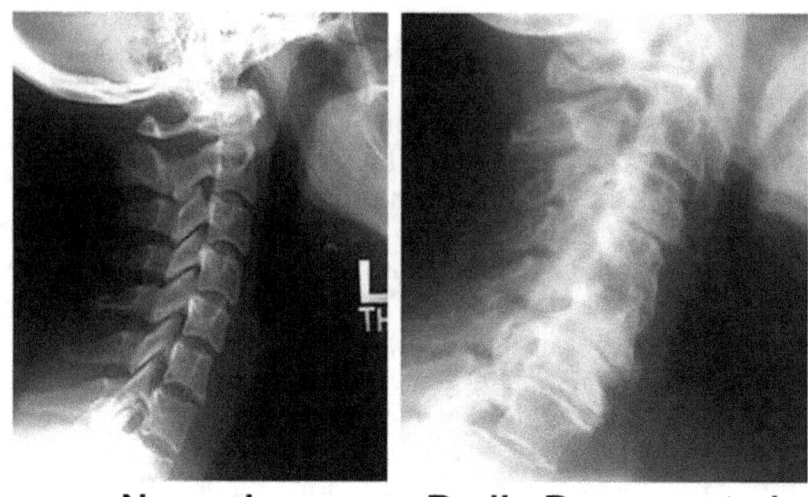

Normal   **Badly Degenerated**

Can you guess who is healthier?

Chiropractors look for bones and joints that aren't moving properly in your spine and frame. When they find a dysfunctional joint, known as a "subluxation," a chiropractor will put a quick force into the joint, known as a chiropractic adjustment, which frees the joint and allows it to function in its proper range of motion. This keeps the joints healthy and allows the nervous system to function at its peak.

Having healthy joints in our spine prevents wear and tear and keeps the shock absorbing discs between our vertebrae hydrated so they can do their job. When you get adjusted regularly you will be more in tune with your body, more relaxed over all, and more aware of how your spine should be functioning.

Please note that when you "crack" your back, this is not the same as being adjusted by a chiropractor. When you crack your own back, the only joints that are "cracking" are the ones already moving properly. You simply don't have the knowledge or skill to find the real dysfunctional joints, or the correct leverage to adjust the joints that are stuck and dysfunctional.

Getting adjusted regularly will reduce the incidence of pain, disc degeneration and back surgery. Chiropractic is not only for the spine. A good chiropractor will check your hips, knees, and ankles to make sure they are in alignment as well. Just like keeping your car's tires in alignment will reduce premature wear, keeping your hips and knees in alignment will minimize wear and tear, promote proper function, and reduce the possibility of requiring hip or knee replacement surgery down the road. According to a study performed by American Specialty Health Plans Inc,[8]:

• Chiropractic care cut the cost of treating back pain by 28%.

• Chiropractic care reduced hospitalizations among back pain patients by 41%.

• Chiropractic care reduced back surgeries by 32%.

• Chiropractic care reduced the cost of medical imaging, such as X-rays or MRIs, by 37%.

It's clear: in order to have a properly functioning spine, it's imperative you get it checked regularly by a chiropractor.

---

[8] Legorreta, Antonio P., R. Douglas Metz, Craig F. Nelson, Saurabh Ray, Helen Oster Chernicoff, and Nicholas A. Dinubile. 2004. "Comparative Analysis of Individuals with and without Chiropractic Coverage: Patient Characteristics, Utilization, and Costs." Archives of Internal Medicine 164 (18): 1985–92. doi:10.1001/archinte.164.18.1985.

It's also critically important to keep your muscles and connective tissue, your skeleton's support system healthy.

Chapter 3: Muscles and connective tissue

Many layers of muscle surround our bones to keep us standing and allow us to move around. Our spine and frame is like an antenna, it should be standing straight up and supported by our muscles, the guy wires that hold us up.

We have deep muscles that run along our spine and connect our vertebrae, which we talked about earlier, another layer of stabilizing muscles that keep us balanced and stable, and superficial muscles that move us around.

Between and throughout these various levels of muscle is a saran-wrap like tissue called fascia, which connects muscle to muscle and muscle to bone. If you've ever cut open a chicken, fascia is the white tissue you may see that surrounds the muscles.

Our muscles are linked together in chains connected to each other in the body. If a muscle becomes dysfunctional due to postural change or injury, it will create a cascade of aberrant function and potential injury.

The biggest cause of damage to our muscles and fascia isn't large catastrophic injury, but repetitive stress injuries. The most common cause of repetitive stress injury in our society is due to constantly sitting.

The Effects of Sitting

Sitting is one of the worst things you can do to your body, yet most of us spend the majority of our time in this position. Since we started school we have been sitting many hours per day. As adults, it's not uncommon to sit 8-10 hours or more daily. We sit to eat breakfast, sit at work, sit at lunch, sit at dinner, then sit on the couch to relax. Unless we are

33

exercising or active for more time than we are sedentary, the effects of sitting are unavoidable.

The effect of all this sitting are two conditions known as upper and lower crossed syndromes. The sitting position causes a pattern of shortening and lengthening in opposing muscle groups which follows a cross pattern in our shoulders and hips.

In upper crossed syndrome, sitting posture along with gravitational pull causes your head and shoulders to inch forward. This position of slumping shoulders and forward head causes your chest muscles and posterior neck muscles to tighten and become shorter. These muscles adapt to their short position and stay short, through a process called "adaptive shortening."

When some muscles get short, their antagonists, or opposite muscles, have to stretch. These stretched muscles become lengthened and weak through a process of "stretch inhibition."

For every one inch of forward head travel, your neck has to support 12-15 more pounds of weight. This extra stress will lead to a chronically tight and stiff neck, causing reduced range of motion, headaches, and premature neck degeneration.

Lower crossed syndrome is similar. Your lower back and hip flexors become short and stay short, while your glutes and abs become stretched, loose and weak. As lower crossed syndrome progresses, the abdominal muscles will lose tone and allow the stomach to protrude. This postural distortion and lack of tone is what prevents many people from achieving a visible abdominal six pack.

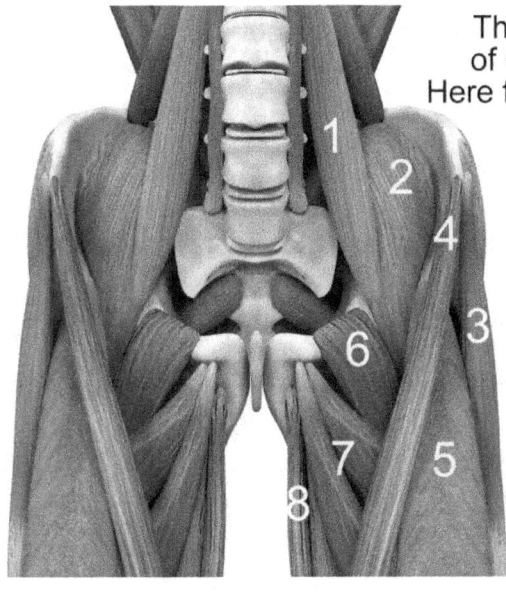

There is a Lot
of Opportunity
Here for Dysfunction

1. Psoas
2. Illiacus
3. Tensor
   Fasciae
   Latae (TFL)
4. Sartorius
5. Quadriceps
   Femoris
6. Pectineus
7. Adductors
8. Gracilis

To make matters worse, without adequate movement, your muscles become stuck to their surrounding tissues and form what are known as adhesions. If you experience an injury such as a muscle strain, scar tissue will form during healing, which will reduce range of motion and create bonds with surrounding tissues. Scar tissue can even be a source of pain, as it has a large number of pain receptors compared to other tissues.

Muscle Injuries

When a muscle is injured, fibroblasts, which are repair cells in the body, lay down collagen to patch up the injured areas. Unfortunately, the body deposits the collagen in a haphazard way, causing the healing muscle to lose elasticity, lose strength and lose ability to fully contract.

Scar tissue can also cause healing muscles or ligaments to stick to surrounding tissues or heal in a misaligned stretched or shortened state. This is why it's important to be adjusted regularly after a sprain/strain injury like whiplash.

Maintaining proper skeletal alignment while your soft tissues heal will allow everything to heal in the right alignment, minimize the injury's impact on your body, and ensure you are able to maintain correct biomechanical function.

These cycles of muscle shortening due to sitting, adhesions, injuries and scar tissue keep our body in a sitting posture even after we are done sitting. The same muscles that are short when we sit stay short when we stand. This pulls our hips forward, causing anterior pelvic tilt and shoulder slump. This wrecks the integrity of our core musculature, and is why our posture progressively worsens as we age.

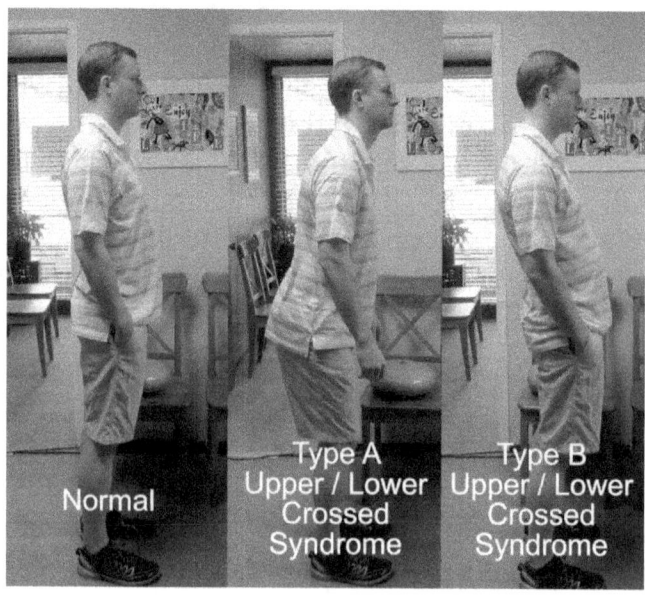

Normal

Type A
Upper / Lower
Crossed
Syndrome

Type B
Upper / Lower
Crossed
Syndrome

Correcting Your Sitting Posture

The correct way to sit to promote proper body mechanics is with your butt all the way back in the chair. If you are looking at a monitor, it should be directly in front of your eyes so your neck can be in a neutral position. Your hips should be at an angle greater than 90 degrees, and your elbows should be bent at a little more than 90 degrees and rest on the keyboard.

If you spend a lot of time at a desk, invest in a nice adjustable desk chair. A nice chair will cost you a few hundred dollars, but if you break the price down to cost per hour, it is only pennies. A local furniture liquidator typically has good deals on slightly used office chairs. My favorite chair is the Herman Miller Embody. The Embody moves with you and is advertised as being health positive, meaning sitting in it makes you healthier. I can sit in my Embody for hours and not get fatigued. Here is an example of proper sitting ergonomics:

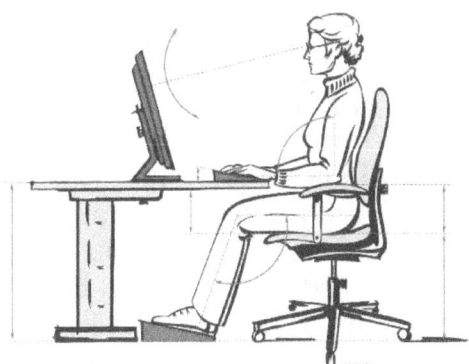

Note the woman is sitting all the way back in the chair, so the chair can adequately support her lumbar curve. Her hips, knees and elbows are bent at 90° or slightly more, the top of the monitor is positioned at eye level, and she sits close enough to the table so her hands rest effortlessly on the keyboard. I like to sit a little more reclined when I work on the computer.

This is the best way to sit, but since you are still in this position for the majority of the day, inevitably your muscles will still begin to adapt. No matter which way you cut it, sitting significantly alters our biomechanics.

An Important Note About Couches

Couches are the worst thing to sit on, unless you have one specifically designed to give you good support, or use a pillow to support your lower back. Most sofas are excessively soft and will cause your lumbar curve to reverse. On the contrary, sitting in a recliner is great. Recliners offer good support, and distribute your weight over more of your body, instead of concentrating your weight onto your lower back. Just make sure to sit in the recliner when it is actually reclined, otherwise it doesn't do much good.

How to Prevent Sitting Disease

To help prevent the harmful effects of sitting, it's critical to move and stretch frequently during the day. Get up and move every 20-30 minutes. Bend, shift, twist and wiggle to get motion into your body. Fidgeting in an uncomfortable chair is a completely normal thing! If you are fidgeting, it probably means you need more frequent breaks to get up and move around. I think it's weird that kids are forced to sit still for so long in school. It might be good for the teachers but it's terrible for the students. Here are a few stretches you can do throughout the day to stretch the muscles shortened when sitting:

Chest Stretch:

Interlace your fingers behind your back, pull your shoulders down and back and pinch your shoulder blades together. You should feel a really good stretch in your chest. Hold this stretch for about 45 seconds to one minute so you feel a good stretch in your chest.

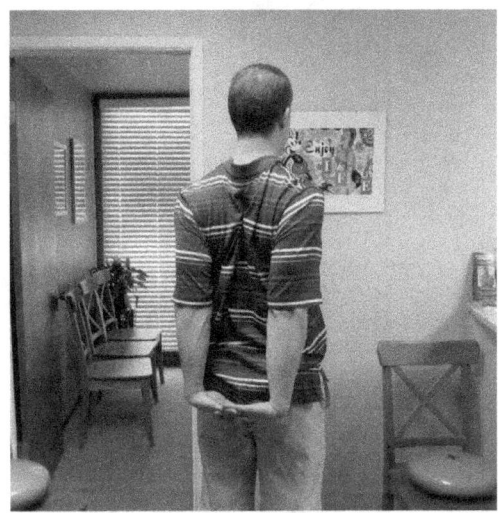

Doorway Stretch:

Go to a doorway and position your arms like the photos below depict, starting with the highest position. Hold each position for 30 seconds. The upper position stretches the front rotator cuff muscle, the subscapularis. The middle position stretches the pec major, and the low position stretches the pec minor.

Both of these stretches are great to do regularly throughout the day. Remember in both these stretches to contract the muscles between your shoulder blades to pinch them together. This will force the stretched muscles to relax and allow them to stretch further.

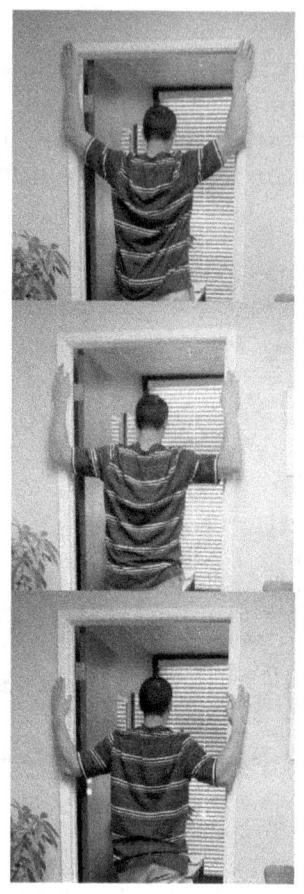

To prevent the effects of sitting on our lower body, I recommend the following three chair stretches that focus on the hip flexors.

Chair Stretches:

The first stretch focuses on the anterior hip muscles and quadriceps. Find a sofa or padded chair, and put one leg behind you so your knee is on the seat and your foot is on the backrest. If you push down on a stick like I am in the picture, your core will be engaged and you will be able to target your anterior hip muscles and quadriceps a little more effectively.

The second stretch focuses on the deep hip flexors including the psoas and illiacus. Make sure to arch your back far so you feel a good stretch deep behind your abs. You can turn away from the stretching leg to increase the stretch. Hold these stretches for 45 seconds each, one right after another, then do the other side

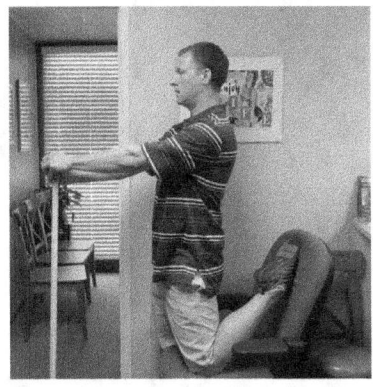

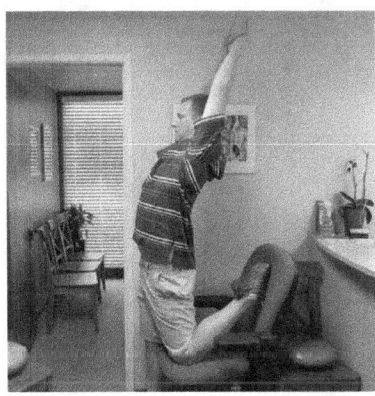

The last stretch for the hip flexors is performed by placing one foot on the seat of a chair, keeping the pelvis neutral and pointed forward, and then leaning into the elevated leg. The stretch should be felt in the front of the hip of the grounded

leg. Squeeze the glute of the ground leg to get even more stretch. This is a great stretch for all muscles that attach to the front of your illium, or pelvic bone.

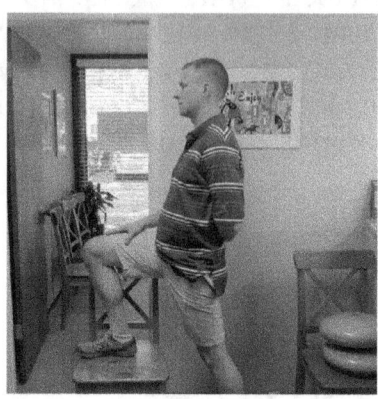

While stretching is important, it is not enough by itself to remedy a serious postural distortion. In this situation the muscles are all stuck together, making it difficult to isolate muscles to stretch individually. The muscles need to be freed from each other in order to function properly.

Correcting a Postural Dysfunction and Maintaining Correct Mechanics

The only effective way to correct upper and lower crossed syndrome or prevent it from occurring, is by keeping your muscle and skeletal system healthy. This entails regular chiropractic visits and deep tissue massage, and resistance training. A chiropractor will help make sure the joints in your spine are aligned and functioning properly, and a qualified massage therapist, specializing in clinical or therapeutic massage, will work on releasing the tight, short and adhered hip flexors including your psoas, illiacus, other hip and lower back muscles.

A good rule of thumb for finding the right massage therapist is to find one working out of a chiropractic or physical therapy office or dedicated sports therapy clinic. It is also worthwhile to get worked on by several therapists so you know the differences in techniques they use and so you find someone that you relate to.

Once you have begun undoing the damage, you are going to want to restore muscle balance to your hips and shoulders. This may take some assistance from a trainer or even some hip and shoulder rehabilitation from a physical therapist if your structural dysfunctions are severe.

At first while you are being adjusted and cared for, you may be instructed just to maintain standing balance on an unstable surface like a wobble board or bosu ball. This retrains your nervous system and your muscles to adopt the correct alignment of your spine and body. Once you are starting to hold the correct alignment you will be shown corrective exercises to strengthen the hips, glutes and core.

First, you will be advised to practice stability and balance by holding static postures, often in a crawl or bridge position. Then, movement will be added to these postures, forcing you to keep your core stable while moving your limbs. To make things more challenging you may be asked to perform these exercises on an unstable surface, like a bosu ball or wobble board.

Eventually weight training will be incorporated into your rehabilitation program.

Regular resistance training with correct form and full range of motion will help break up muscular adhesions and ensure your muscles are moving on each other. If you are new, consult with a personal trainer. Find a trainer who has a successful private studio of their own. I advise to start with light weights and higher repetitions. Perform exercises that strengthen the lengthened and stretched muscles of your upper back and glutes. Use machines at first and as you become more sophisticated move to free weights and more compound movements like bench presses, pull ups and squats and deadlifts.

Please note that it takes time and significant effort to rehabilitate years of developing dysfunction from sitting and injury, but as someone who suffered from postural and stability issues myself, I can tell you that the end result of working correctly is well worth the effort. A proper functioning body and core will help you look better and pay HUGE dividends in functioning properly and in avoiding injury down the road.

Lifting

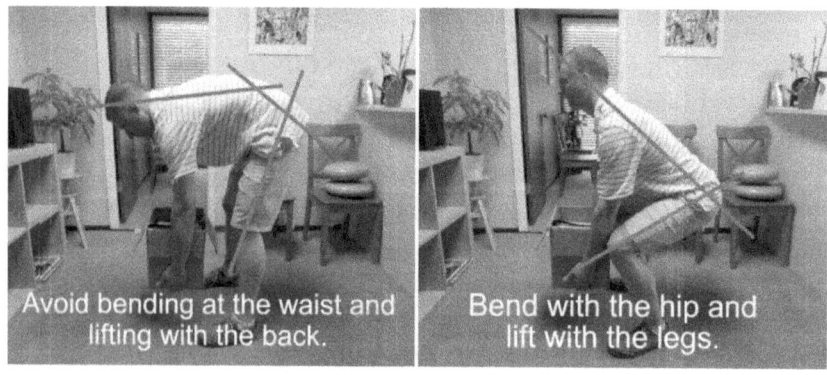

Avoid bending at the waist and lifting with the back.

Bend with the hip and lift with the legs.

Our back muscles, along with the rest of our core (yes back muscles are part of your core), are meant to work as stabilizers to keep our spine straight and balanced. Our legs are designed to work as our prime movers for moving and lifting. To lift with your legs, it's necessary to keep your back and core rigid, while your legs bend and maneuver you into a position to lift. Lifting with your legs involves bending at the hip. Lifting with the back involves bending at the waist and using the back muscles to extend a flexed spine, which can cause injury.

Hip Hinge

In some fitness circles the "hip hinge" is a big buzzword, and for good reason. Training the proper use of the hip hinge is great practice for lifting anything out there. Hip hinge means we bend at the hips like a hinge, and not at the waist. A deep squat requires proper mechanics and function of our core and hips. One way to see how your core and hips are working together, and to experience the sensation of using your legs for movement and core for stability, is to hold a stick or pvc pipe behind your back with your arms while you perform a squat or deadlift.

The key here is to have the stick contact three points, the back of your head, your mid/upper back, and hips. When in this position, practice squatting or bending with your hips as you would to lift something from the ground. If you can't do these movements without losing contact with the stick, your spine and joint mechanics need rehabilitation.

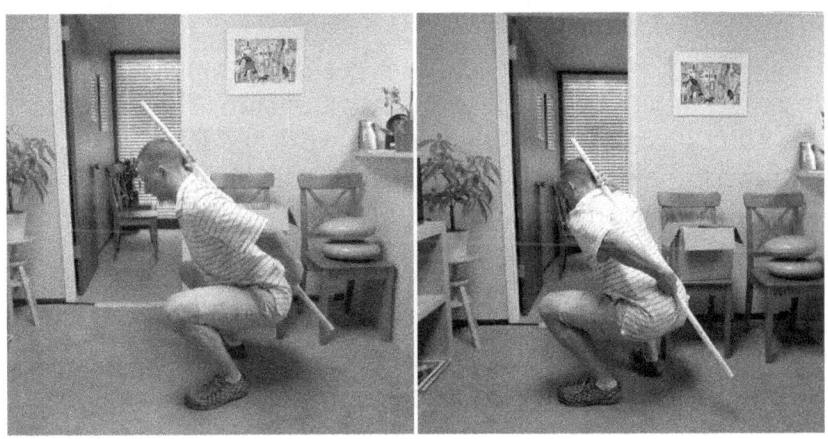

The Core

What is the core anyway? The core is made up of all the muscles that connect the spine, pelvis and rib cage, including the lower back muscles.

When training the core, it's vital to train the individual muscles in context with the rest of the core, so the muscles are all being engaged. This is why sit-ups are the worst type of exercise to perform when training the core.

The abdominal muscles, in their purest function, are meant to resist spinal extension, the backwards bending of the spine. When doing sit-ups, the abs are being used to create spinal flexion. In a sit up, the abs might be used for the first two inches of movement, but the actual sitting up portion of the movement is performed by the hip flexors. This is an ineffective and counterproductive way to train the abs.

Most people suffer from some degree of lower and upper crossed syndromes. In lower crossed syndrome, the hip flexors are chronically tight and short, and the abs are stretched and weak. Performing traditional sit-ups just encourages this imbalance.

The best way to train the abs is to get them to perform their designed function: resisting spinal extension. The secret to training the abs, is that you want to work them in conjunction with the hip flexors, but in a stabilizing role, so both are being used to perform their respective function. They are working together, yet independently.

All the muscles should be performing their specific role in context with the rest of the muscles. Here's what I mean: The core should be activated all around and always kept tight and rigid to stabilize the trunk, while the leg muscles perform the gross movements, either moving the legs, or moving the trunk. The core should always be tight when doing any type of movement.

Some of the best type of exercises to work the abs that utilize many core muscles include leg lifts while hanging from a bar, leg lifts using a roman chair, flutter kicks, flutter kicks on a swiss ball, and leg lifts.

All these exercises encourage movement of the hip flexors and extensors independently of core movement. Training the core specifically is a little different than training the abs. The job of your core is to transfer power between the lower and upper body, and to provide stability. To train the core in its entirety, the best type of exercises, naturally, are exercises that involve power transmission between the lower and upper body. Compound movements like squats and deadlifts, overhead squats, olympic lifts and rotational movements in the transverse plane like throwing, and swinging are all great exercises to do. For the untrained, I recommend consulting with someone who can give you some instruction in these lifts, as they are very complex and difficult to master.

In summary, here's where we are so far:

Your central nervous system is your body's central processing unit, and is responsible for all its function. Stressors in our environment, including emotional, chemical and physical stress change the way our nervous system interprets and responds to its environment. Stress affects our immune system, our mental health, and our musculoskeletal system. Stress can interfere with your body's natural healing ability and create postural changes that lead to premature wear and tear and significant physical dysfunction.

Chiropractic, along with deep tissue massage and exercise can keep your infrastructure functioning at its peak.

Structural problems don't happen overnight. The solution might take months, but is necessary, because bad posture does more than just make us look bad or ruin our biomechanics. Bad posture can seriously compromise the function of our heart and lungs.

Chapter 4: Heart and Lungs

Your heart and lungs are intimately connected. These two organs work together to make sure every part of the body gets the oxygen and nutrients it needs. The lungs oxygenate the blood, and the heart pumps it through the body. Bad posture handicaps these systems from working properly by reducing the size of your thoracic cavity and decreasing the amount of space for your heart and lungs to do their job.

Blood returns from your body to the heart through veins. Your veins don't have much pressure in them, and the primary way blood is pumped back to the heart is through movement of skeletal muscles (another reason to stay moving). Your venous system culminates with two large veins, the inferior and superior vena cava, that dump deoxygenated blood into the heart.

Returning blood is deposited into a chamber in the heart called the right atrium. It passes through the tricuspid valve into the right ventricle, where it is propelled into the lungs for oxygenation. Having a reduced chest size prevents the lungs from expanding to their full capacity. If you can't breathe deeply to get the oxygen you need, you'll have to breathe faster. This significantly limits your capacity for exertion.

After oxygenation the blood returns to the heart's left atrium, is pumped through the mitral valve into the left ventricle, where it is then shot like a geyser through the aortic valve and into the aorta. The aorta splits into other arteries that supply our organs and tissues, including our heart, with oxygen and nutrients.

If you have a smaller chest cavity due to bad posture, the heart and your elastic arteries will be squeezed and have less room to expand. This increased pressure will reduce stroke volume, the amount of blood sent per heartbeat, and increase blood pressure. This will create an increased resting heart rate, and ultimately limit the amount of blood our heart can pump to our body.

About 2000 gallons of blood moves through the heart per day, but none of this blood actually supplies the heart itself. The heart muscle gets its blood and nutrients through the coronary arteries, the first arteries that branch off from the aorta. The heart is always working and needs a continuous supply of blood to properly function. When the heart doesn't get the blood it needs, usually because of a blockage of these arteries, the result is a myocardial infarction or a heart attack.

The papillary muscles in your heart control the opening and closing of our heart valves. When our heart beats, blood is pumped through these valves. After every beat, these valves close to prevent blood from flowing backwards. When the papillary muscles don't get the blood they need, they can malfunction and allow blood to flow backwards. This is known as regurgitation and can be heard as a heart murmur.

Ensuring good posture by maintaining a properly functioning skeletal structure and muscle system will massively benefit you later in life, as will following the rules outlined in the next section.

Top Three Rules for Respiratory and Cardiovascular Health

First rule: Exercise. Use It or Lose It

Your heart is meant to pump blood and your lungs are meant to breathe. Let them work! Your body needs oxygen, and your heart needs exercise like every other muscle in your body. Aerobic exercise has been shown to reduce coronary artery disease, blood lipid levels and blood pressure. Plus, it will make you feel good! Aerobic exercise reduces stress and can help alleviate depression and anxiety. Further, it can help fight diabetes and aging. Your heart and lungs are meant to be used, so use them!

When your lungs expand fully and your breathing muscles are fully utilized, you will increase lung capacity, breathe more deeply and have a lower respiratory rate. Untrained individuals and those with poor posture lose their ability to inhale deeply, and are forced to fulfill their oxygen requirement by increasing their rate of respiration, ultimately limiting their capacity for physical performance and proper function.

Regular cardiovascular exercise will promote lower blood pressure, lower resting heart rate, and increase the capacity of our heart to function properly through stressful situations.

Keeping Your Heart Healthy Through Exercise

According to the American Heart Association, for maximum cardiovascular and respiratory benefit, you should strive to keep your heart beating between 50-85% of its maximum rate when exercising for general health.

The most widely accepted formula for maximum heart rate calculation is:

$HRmax = 220 - age$

A better, more accurate and more recent formula is:

$HRmax = 208 - (0.7 \times age)$

The best way to figure out your maximum heart rate is by undergoing a cardiac stress test administered by a doctor, but for most people these calculations will be acceptable.

This zone keeps your body in a state of aerobic metabolism, which means your body is using fat and oxygen as its source of energy. Above this aerobic range is the anaerobic range, which has higher energy demands, and is only sustainable for short bursts of activity.

Basic health guidelines dictate that everybody participate in aerobic exercise for 30 minutes per session, five days per week, but regular vigorous exercise even for as little as ten minutes has shown to significantly increase heart health.

For new trainees, the AHA recommends to start on the low end of the target heart rate range. People experienced with exercise may find the upper range most appropriate.

Generally, your heart rate should be kept in this zone for the entire duration of the exercise. If you have to stop to catch your breath, you are stepping into the anaerobic zone. Please consult your physician before beginning any new exercise program.

Second rule: Avoid Tobacco Products

Everybody knows smoking ruins your health, but really, in addition to the carcinogens in the smoke, nicotine is also a killer! Smoking and nicotine are responsible for the two leading causes of death in the US: heart disease and cancer.

Nicotine, previously thought just to be the addictive component in tobacco, has also been shown to contribute to heart disease. Electronic cigarettes are NOT a safe alternative to tobacco. They still have nicotine!

This addictive drug hardens your arteries. Nicotine stimulates the smooth muscle around your arteries to grow into the endothelium, the innermost layer of your blood vessels. When the muscle starts poking through the vessel walls, the body interprets this as damage, and will increase your levels of low density lipoproteins (LDLs), somewhat erroneously known as bad cholesterol (to be explained in the upcoming section on fat), to try to patch up the damage with cholesterol and plaque.

Another component of cigarette smoke, acroline, actually inhibits cholesterol metabolism. This will result in higher cholesterol levels and more opportunity for plaque deposits and arterial stiffening. All of this arterial stiffening will drive up blood pressure and stress the heart. Additionally, the increased plaque buildups can sometimes rupture and form a blood clot.

Blood clots can block blood flow to the heart and cause a heart attack. They may even dislodge and travel to the lungs or brain, causing a pulmonary embolism or stroke. Both these situations can cause severe incapacitation, disability or death.

Cigarette smoking causes 90% of lung cancers. Over 7000 chemicals exist in tobacco smoke, and of these, at least 70 are known carcinogens.[9] These compounds affect our bodies with each puff. Carcinogens alter DNA structure and cause mutations, while other chemicals, known as tumor promoters, prevent the body from controlling normal cell growth.[10]

---

[9] "CDC - What Are the Risk Factors for Lung Cancer?" 2014. Accessed August 26. http://www.cdc.gov/cancer/lung/basic_info/risk_factors.htm.

Nicotine also can stimulate angiogenesis, or the formation of new blood vessels, which can provide blood to growing tumors.

Third rule: Follow an Anti Inflammatory Diet

Contrary to prevailing common thought, eating fat and cholesterol doesn't necessarily make you fat or clog your arteries. In fact, eating the right kinds of fats can be very beneficial.

Sugar and carbohydrates are the cause of heart disease, not fats.

High levels of cholesterol and triglycerides due to genetic factors or chronic disease might warrant management with your medical doctor, but generally, drugs are not always necessary for slightly elevated cholesterol levels.

Blocking cholesterol with statin drugs has deleterious effects on our chemistry. One negative side effect includes preventing the production of coenzyme Q10 (CoQ10), a substance vital to proper heart function. CoQ10 deficiency has been linked to many diseases including heart failure, and it is often used as a treatment for people with heart failure.

Statin drugs can also cause muscle pain, muscle cramps and occasionally even muscle breakdown, known as

---

[10] Centers for Disease Control and Prevention (US); National Center for Chronic Disease Prevention and Health Promotion (US); Office on Smoking and Health (US). How Tobacco Smoke Causes Disease: The Biology and Behavioral Basis for Smoking-Attributable Disease: A Report of the Surgeon General. Atlanta (GA): Centers for Disease Control and Prevention (US); 2010. 5, Cancer. Available from: http://www.ncbi.nlm.nih.gov/books/NBK53010/

rhabdomyolosis, which can lead to kidney failure and even death.

If you have slightly elevated cholesterol, rather than jumping right to drugs, take a good look at your diet first. In past decades, fats have been blamed for arteriosclerosis, heart disease, and other indicators of poor health, but now research shows that fats are not all bad, and some are even very healthy.

Fats are an important part of your body and your diet. Fats are involved in cell membrane structural integrity, production of necessary enzymes for metabolic pathways, they keep your brain, eyes and heart healthy, can lower systemic inflammation, and more.

Chapter 5: Diet

Fat

There are three main types of fat molecules: phospholipids, cholesterol and triglycerides. Cholesterol and triglycerides are the most relevant fats in our conversation here.

Cholesterol is a vital part of our body. It makes up a critical part of our cells' membrane, and is a precursor to important steroid hormones. Cholesterol in itself is not inherently bad. In fact, it's not really bad at all. The reason cholesterol gets a bad rap is for its role in tissue healing.

After eating a meal of sugar or simple carbohydrates, your blood sugar spikes. High levels of blood sugar puts undue stress on the endothelium, the inside layer of your blood vessels.

This damage creates systemic inflammation. High blood sugar also reduces the formation of nitrous oxide (NO), the molecule responsible for relaxing our arteries.

Systemic inflammation and arterial damage leads the body to increase cholesterol levels in order to heal and repair. This combination of vessel damage, cholesterol and plaque accumulation in damaged areas, and the inability of our arteries to relax, all add up to stiffer arteries.

High cholesterol is not the cause of heart disease, but merely an indicator of an unhealthy lifestyle.

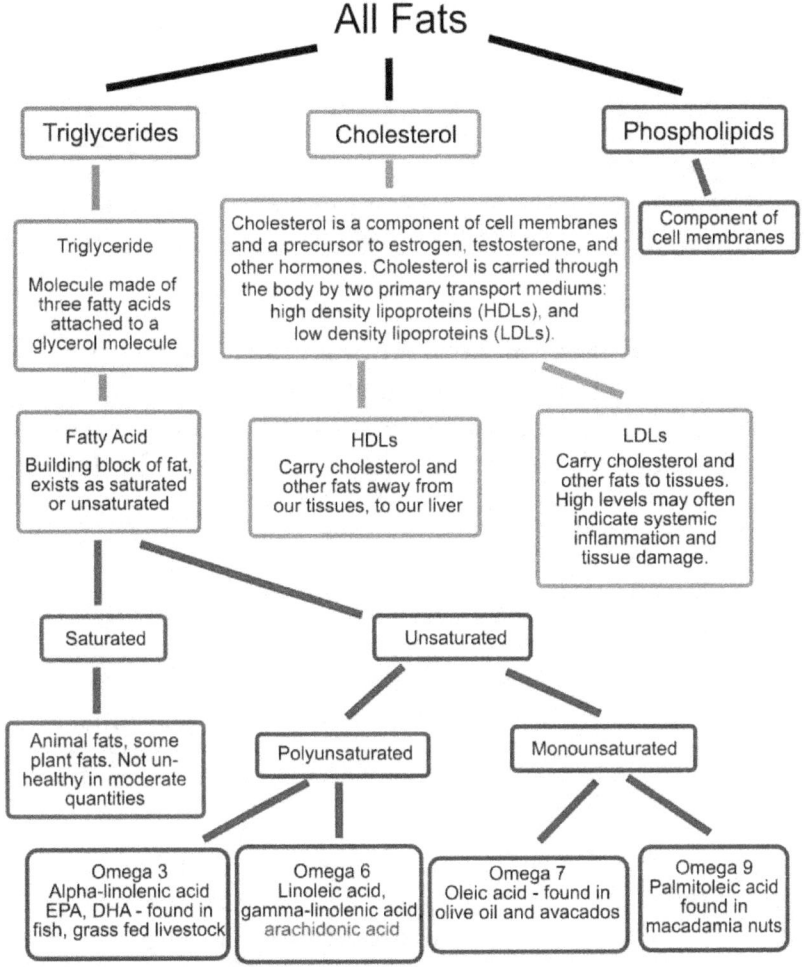

When your arteries get damaged or inflamed, cholesterol is sent to patch up the damaged area. LDLs, or low density lipoproteins, act as a transport mechanism or container to carry cholesterol and other fats around the body in response to inflammation. When the LDL reaches the damaged area, it binds to the damaged tissue to release cholesterol for tissue repair.

LDLs are not necessarily bad and LDLs are not a risk factor themselves; high levels of LDLs are an indicator of systemic inflammation or tissue damage. Consuming large amounts of fat will elevate blood cholesterol and triglyceride levels, so don't use this information as a free pass to eat all the fat you want.

What we generally think of as fats, like the fat enumerated in foods' nutritional information label, are known chemically as triglycerides. A triglyceride is a combination of a glycerol molecule attached to three fatty acids. In triglyceride form, fats may be transported throughout the body for used or storage.

Fatty acids are small building blocks of fat. In their free form, not attached to other molecules, they are known as free fatty acids (FFAs). FFAs are a very important energy source, and are generally the preferred energy source for most muscle because their metabolism yields the most cellular energy (ATP).

There are two primary types of fatty acids, saturated and unsaturated. A fatty acid is "saturated" when every one of its carbon atoms is bonded to the maximum amount of hydrogen atoms possible. "Unsaturated" fatty acids have carbon molecules that are double bonded to their neighboring carbon atoms, and therefore can't accept the maximum possible number of hydrogen atoms.

Saturated fats are found in high levels in animal fat products including cheese, butter, lard and fatty meat. Saturated fat is also found in coconut oil, palm oil and chocolate. In a flawed study where data manipulation dictated the findings, saturated fat was found to be linked to heart disease. This, of course, led to mania about saturated fat. Marketers exploited this mania and started producing partially hydrogenated oils, their "healthy" alternative to saturated fat.

In order to create more "favorable" chemical properties to mimic lard and butter, unsaturated fats in liquid form like vegetable oil were hydrogenated, or reacted to accept more hydrogen. Hydrogenating oils makes them solid at room temperature and increases their shelf life. Margarine and Crisco are examples of hydrogenated oils. They were marketed as being healthy, yet contained trans fat, a very unhealthy component.

Trans fats are uncommon in nature, and are formed as a byproduct during the hydrogenation process. "Trans" refers to a chemical structural designation. Trans fat have been shown to significantly increase inflammation levels in the body, increase LDL levels, and damage arteries.[11] Only recently have we realized that hydrogenated oils and their associated trans fats were bad for you.

Unfortunately, the stigma of saturated fat remains, despite recent studies showing that saturated fat intake is not associated with an increased risk of coronary heart disease or cardiovascular disease.[12] Some other studies have shown that when a portion of dietary saturated fat is replaced with polyunsaturated fat, there is a slight health benefit, although this is likely due to the anti-inflammatory nature of many

[11] Mozaffarian, Dariush, Tobias Pischon, Susan E. Hankinson, Nader Rifai, Kaumudi Joshipura, Walter C. Willett, and Eric B. Rimm. 2004. "Dietary Intake of Trans Fatty Acids and Systemic Inflammation in Women." The American Journal of Clinical Nutrition 79 (4): 606–12.
[12] Siri-Tarino, Patty W, Qi Sun, Frank B Hu, and Ronald M Krauss. 2010. "Meta-Analysis of Prospective Cohort Studies Evaluating the Association of Saturated Fat with Cardiovascular disease12345." The American Journal of Clinical Nutrition 91 (3): 535–46. doi:10.3945/ajcn.2009.27725.

polyunsaturated fats, and not to a decrease in saturated fat consumption.

Unsaturated fat is broken down into two categories: monounsaturated (MUFA) and polyunsaturated (PUFA). This naming refers to how many carbon double bonds exist within the fatty acid. MUFAs have one double bond (mono), and PUFAs have two or more (poly). The Omega fatty acids (Omega 3, 6, 7, 9) are all unsaturated fats and all, with one notable exception, have anti-inflammatory properties.

Monounsaturated fats include oleic acid (omega 9) and palmitoleic acid (omega 7). Large amounts of oleic acid are found in olive oil, almonds and avocados. Palmitoleic acid, the essential fatty acid, is found in macadamia nuts.

Polyunsaturated fats are the famous omega 3 and 6 fatty acids you probably (hopefully) have heard about. The three omega 3 fatty acids are alpha-linolenic acid, an essential fatty acid, and the two healthy fatty acids found in fish, EPA (eicosapentaenoic acid) and DHA (docosahexaenoic acid).

These two fish oils, EPA and DHA, have incredibly beneficial properties for cardiovascular and neurological health. EPA lowers systemic inflammation levels and improves cardiovascular health. DHA too helps improve cardiovascular health and also boosts mental function. DHA deficiency may play a role in cognitive decline, and DHA supplementation has been shown to improve learning and memory function in patients with Alzheimer's.[13]

---

[13] Yurko-Mauro, Karin, Deanna McCarthy, Dror Rom, Edward B. Nelson, Alan S. Ryan, Andrew Blackwell, Norman Salem, and Mary Stedman. 2010. "Beneficial Effects of Docosahexaenoic Acid on Cognition in Age-Related Cognitive Decline." Alzheimer's & Dementia: The Journal of the Alzheimer's Association 6 (6): 456–64. doi:10.1016/j.jalz.2010.01.013.

There are three omega 6 fatty acids: linoleic, the essential fatty acid, gamma-linolenic, and arachidonic.

Omega 6 : 3 Ratio

Despite needing omega 6 fatty acids in our diet, one of them, arachadonic acid (AA), has negative inflammatory properties. In a healthy diet, the anti-inflammatory properties of omega 3s will directly counteract the inflammation brought on by AA. The problem is, most western diets have WAY MORE omega 6 content than omega 3 content.

A healthy diet has an O6:O3 ratio of 4:1 or less. The average western diet has a ratio of 11:1 to 30:1! This ratio frequently is attributed to fatty processed foods, fried food, cooking oil and red meat.

Most cooking oil has a very high O6:O3 ratio. Oils high in this ratio include sunflower, safflower, corn and peanut, all with little to virtually no omega 3 content. Grass fed butter, with a nearly 1:1 ratio, and coconut oil are good alternatives.

Omega 6:3 Ratios in Cooking Oils (Predominantly PUFAs):

Canola Oil	2:1
Safflower Oil	Virtually no Omega 3
Sunflower Oil	18:1 to 200:1
Olive Oil	13:1
Soybean Oil	7.5:1
Cottonseed Oil	Virtually No Omega 3
Peanut Oil	No Omega 3
Flaxseed Oil	1:4

Red meat traditionally has a moderately high O6:O3 ratio. Grain fed beef, according to one study, averages 7.65:1, and grass fed 1.53:1, making grass fed beef healthy and good to eat![14]

When it comes to pork, stick with wild boar, as one study found the O6:O3 ratio in wild boar they examined to be 3:1, and the ratio in commercially farmed pigs was very high, with virtually no O3 content.[15] According to these numbers, free range pigs might be expected to have a more favorable ratio than commercially farmed pigs.

Quick guidelines to consuming fats:

• Cholesterol is good for you — our body uses it to repair tissue damage and as a precursor to steroid hormones

• LDLs are not "bad," they are a cholesterol transport mechanism our body uses to repair itself. When your LDL levels are high, it's usually in response to damage taking place in your body.

• Animal fats aren't bad to eat. If the animal has been fed its intended diet, its fats are healthy. That being said, don't go overboard.

• Processed food, fast food and fried food generally have high levels of unhealthy inflammatory fats.

---

[14] Daley, Cynthia A, Amber Abbott, Patrick S Doyle, Glenn A Nader, and Stephanie Larson. 2010. "A Review of Fatty Acid Profiles and Antioxidant Content in Grass-Fed and Grain-Fed Beef." *Nutrition Journal* 9 (March): 10. doi:10.1186/1475-2891-9-10.

[15] Fine, L.-B., and B. C. Davidson. 2008. "Comparison of Lipid and Fatty Acid Profiles of Commercially Raised Pigs with Laboratory Pigs and Wild-Ranging Warthogs." *South African Journal of Science* 104 (7-8): 314–16.

• EPA and DHA, naturally occurring oils found in fish, are amazingly good for you.

Carbs

Unless you are following a strict ketogenic diet, which is fairly difficult to maintain for extended periods of time, our body and brain need carbs.

Sure, some endurance athletes follow a ketogenic diet, but they are very careful to keep their body in an aerobic state, where the body uses fat and oxygen to make energy. Doing any high intensity exercise on a diet like this will leave you huffing and puffing and depleted of energy. Plus for me, being limited in my diet isn't something I'm interested in. I like having the flexibility to eat anything I want, and if you are exercising regularly, you should be able to as well.

When considering carbs in your diet, it's important to consider their effect on your physiology, specifically their impact on your blood sugar. We previously mentioned that high blood sugar can cause endothelial stress and inflammation, so it's important to keep your blood sugar from spiking. The best way to do this is to become familiar with the glycemic index of the various carbs you consume.

Glycemic Index

A food's glycemic index indicates how fast something you eat turns into blood sugar. Of course, the faster your food turns into sugar, the worse it is to eat. The reason is this: if your blood sugar spikes and you don't use that sugar as energy, a lot of it will be stored as fat.

Insulin is responsible for turning blood sugar into stored energy. Insulin turns blood sugar into glycogen and triglycerides. Glycogen is stored in the muscle and liver, and is quickly converted back to sugar when we begin exercising or our blood sugar drops too low. Triglycerides are stored in fat cells.

We are born with a finite number of fat cells. The more triglycerides you try to cram into these fat cells, the larger they become. Eventually they get so big that your body chemistry changes and you develop insulin resistance. This results in a metabolic disorder known as type 2 diabetes.

The glycemic index is rated on a scale of 100. 100 is the rating of pure sugar, glucose. Every food is scored in relation to glucose. The higher the food rates, the faster it will raise blood sugar.

Now, another metric you should be aware of besides glycemic index is a food's glycemic load.

Glycemic load is a food's effect on blood sugar based on the amount of carbohydrates consumed.

Every one unit of a food's glycemic load equals the effect of eating one gram of pure glucose.

For example, watermelon has a high glycemic index of 72. However, it's mostly water. If you eat a 100 gram serving you are really only eating about 5 grams of carbohydrates. The formula for finding glycemic load is:

[(grams of carbohydrates per serving)*(glycemic index)] / 100

This makes the glycemic load of watermelon 3.6. Therefore, if you eat 100 grams of watermelon, it will affect your blood sugar the same as 3.6 grams of pure sugar, making it a decent treat.

On the contrary, the real culprits are the dense starchy carbohydrates like bagels, pasta and white potatoes. Generally, it's best to minimize the consumption of these types of carbs, especially bagels which are particularly dense, but combining them with other food groups will mitigate their blood spiking characteristics.

Outcome Based Eating vs Performance Based Eating

The bottom line is that you should eat for your goals. If you are overweight and want to lose some weight, the best thing to do is to get on a ketogenic diet and incorporate an exercise regimen. There are many schools of thought as to what kind of exercise to incorporate, however you cannot go wrong with weight training along with aerobic exercise like brisk walks for about an hour. Invest in yourself and consult with a personal training studio for best results.

If your goals are building muscle or excelling at sports or competition, you are going to want to incorporate carbohydrates into your diet. Your body burns sugar during anaerobic (high intensity) exercise, and needs carbohydrates about an hour before and immediately after exercise to replenish glycogen, the stored fuel in our muscles and liver.

Add Fat, Lower Glycemic Index.

Fats slow digestion. When you eat fat, it stimulates CCK, a substance involved with coordinating digestion. CCK stimulates the production of fat digesting bile, and slows the movement of food from your stomach to your intestines so the bile has adequate time to do its job. Fats therefore slow down the digestion process, preventing rapid blood sugar spikes.

Although study results have been somewhat inconclusive, there is evidence that eating protein can also slow gastric emptying.

I don't necessarily advocate eating carbs and fats together by themselves, but together with other foods in a balanced meal. If you want great approach to combining macronutrients, I highly recommend Dr. John Berardi's work at http://www.precisionnutrition.com

Avoid fruit juice and drinks sweetened with high fructose corn syrup. Fructose has a glycemic index of approximately 19. Sounds good right? Well, it's not. Fructose, unlike other sugars, does not stimulate insulin release. Like we mentioned earlier, insulin regulates blood sugar. Fructose is not regulated by insulin and is metabolized primarily by the liver, where it forms glycerol, a building block of triglycerides.

Fructose will therefore elevate blood triglyceride levels as well as cholesterol levels, particularly low density lipoproteins (LDLs) commonly referred to as "bad cholesterol." High blood triglyceride levels have been linked to atherosclerosis and heart disease. The best guideline to follow for minimizing fructose consumption is: eliminate sweet drinks from your diet including sodas and fruit juices. The stuff will skyrocket your blood sugar.

It's All About Context

Eat carbohydrates in combination with fat and protein to help prevent blood sugar spikes and promote a healthy body and waistline.

Some Dietary Warnings

If you are trying to lose weight, you may want to even cut back on the amount of fruit you eat. If you are eating a ton of fruit and not exercising, be aware that the fruit's sugar is turning into triglycerides and being stored as fat.

If you are into blending and making green smoothies, be conscious of how much fruit you are adding to the smoothie. Don't blend and drink more fruit than you would eat in any one sitting. You may be just getting a lot of sugar instead of a healthy balanced vegetable rich power drink. The same goes for fruit juice like orange juice and the "healthy" juices like pomegranate juice. A good rule of thumb is not to drink more juice than you would get eating the actual fruit.

One thing I see that especially chaps my hide is when I see little kids and toddlers being fed juice like it's supposed to be healthy. There really is a ton of sugar in those "healthy" fruit juices for their small bodies. Go by the same fruit juice rule of thumb for your children. Don't let them drink more juice than they'd get in the equivalent amount of fruit. A whole large orange only produces maybe two ounces of juice, so keep that in mind.

Vegetables are of course very healthy, and I recommend you eat as many servings of veggies as you can, at least one serving with every meal. Vegetables have important anti-oxidants, crucial in preventing cell damage from free radicals.

Cell Aging and Frcc Radicals

One ways "aging" occurs is through shortening of your telomeres.

Telomeres are protective end caps of your chromosomes, the DNA containing structures within most your cells that contain the information necessary to create new cells.

When your chromosomes split and create copies of themselves during cell division, they lose a bit of information from their ends; they become shorter with every duplication. Telomeres, the "end caps" of your chromosomes, are like the hard plastic caps of your shoe laces, these end caps are the part of your chromosomes that become shorter with every duplication.

The telomeres prevent "fraying" of your chromosomes when they are duplicated. It's during this phase of cell duplication, mitosis, where mutations can occur.

It's therefore in your interest to keep your telomeres as long as possible, and scientists look at their length to determine how old you are on a molecular level. There are even tests available to determine the length of your telomeres.

Telomeres are very susceptible to oxidative stress, the impact that free radicals have on your cells, which is why anti-oxidants are good to have in your diet.

Oxidative stress has been shown to play a role in many other diseases including virtually all inflammatory diseases, heart disease, stroke, atherosclerosis, AIDS, neurological disorders like Alzheimer's and Parkinson's and many others.[16]

In a study in the British Journal of Nutrition, researchers found that elderly men who drank three or more cups of tea per day had longer telomeres than men who drank less than

[16] Lobo, V., A. Patil, A. Phatak, and N. Chandra. 2010. "Free Radicals, Antioxidants and Functional Foods: Impact on Human Health." *Pharmacognosy Reviews* 4 (8): 118–26. doi:10.4103/0973-7847.70902.

one cup, and the extra length accounted for a difference of approximately five fewer years of aging.[17]

The most popular tea the men drank was green tea, followed by white oolong tea.

It's critical to include anti-oxidants in your diet. The commonly regarded most important anti-oxidant is glutathione. Glutathione is naturally produced in your body for protection, however as you age less and less is produced.[18]

The best sources for glutathione include raw fresh fruits, raw fresh vegetables, especially cruciferous veggies like broccoli, kale, cauliflower, cabbage, raw milk, undenatured whey protein, meats and egg yolks.

Other foods to eat for their anti-oxidant content include milk thistle, vitamins C, E and D, selenium, alpha lipoic acid, and spices like turmeric, cumin and curcumin.

---

[17] "Cambridge Journals Online - British Journal of Nutrition - Abstract - Chinese Tea Consumption Is Associated with Longer Telomere Length in Elderly Chinese Men." 2015. Accessed February 26. http://journals.cambridge.org/action/displayAbstract;jsessionid=DCB31EE76B4 EB0872242C59D37FAB531.journals?aid=6889032&fileId=S000711450999138 3&inf_contact_key=21f59682852ababf53de745f8b5766179834c61530dead377 31cb69a537137d7.

[18] "Age-Related Changes in the Glutathione Redox System. - PubMed - NCBI." 2015. Accessed February 26. http://www.ncbi.nlm.nih.gov/pubmed/11835271.

Conclusion

The human body is the most amazing piece of precision machinery we could ever hope to own. It's up to us to keep ourselves healthy. If we want to still be active and thriving into our golden years, it's vital we learn about our amazing bodies and how to keep these amazing machines healthy and functioning properly.

Hopefully this guide has shown you a bit about how to care for it.

About the Author

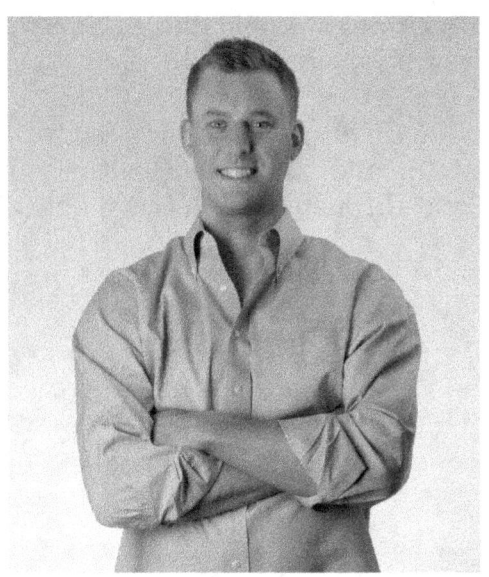

Dr. Alex is a chiropractor specializing in boosting the performance of your high performance body. Whether you are interested in reconditioning your body and creating an athletic foundation to build from, or squeezing out every last bit of performance from your high performance machine, Dr. Alex can help you.

Visit Dr. Alex's practice website for more information: http://www.WiantHealth.com

As an eclectic and hobby heavy individual, in his spare time Alex enjoys playing golf, shooting pool, working out, being outdoors, following boxing and Formula 1, his favorite sports, and doing lots of other cool stuff.

Bonus Audio and Video

I've made a companion audiobook with commentary just for people who purchased my book, that goes into a little more detail about everything presented here.

Additionally, I have two special reports to give you, "5 Keys to a Pain Free Life," and "The Peak Health Formula," along with my "10 Point Ultimate Health Cheat Sheet."

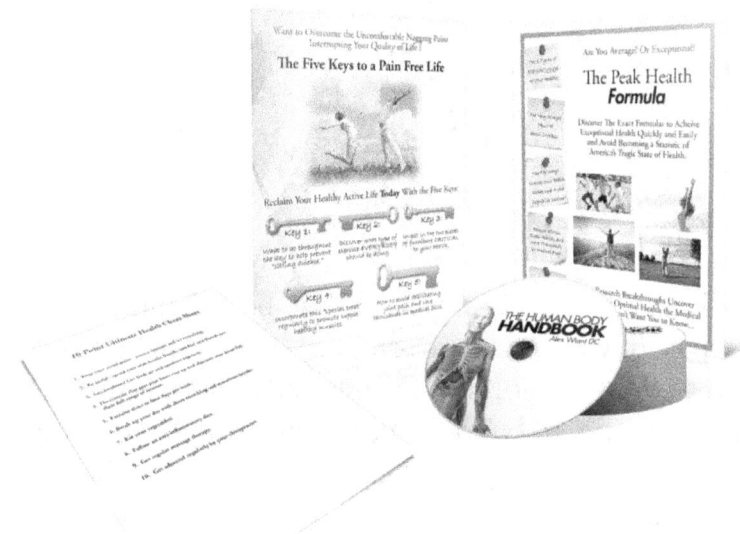

These reports and bonuses include actionable information you can immediately use to significantly improve your health and function

To claim your bonuses, please go to:

http://www.AlexWiant.com/bookbonus

www.ingramcontent.com/pod-product-compliance
Lightning Source LLC
Chambersburg PA
CBHW070607290526
45790CB00002B/822